SUPERFOODS

Eat Right for a Great Life

MICHELE BRITT

Table of Contents

Introduction

Welcome to the Optimized Life! Discover how you are only a few simple steps away from living the life of your dreams. Learn how to achieve anything you can dream with the revolutionary Optimized Living system. This book shows you how easy it is to take the first step through making a few simple changes in your diet!

Are you tired of just surviving life? Do you look around wondering why some people seem to have "it all" going for them? Enjoying a great career . . . an ideal family life . . . and extreme health?

You may think they've been born under a lucky star or with a silver spoon in their mouth. But the fact of the matter is, they've learned the secrets of Optimized Living. Optimized Living gives you the best of all worlds. It takes your life from so-so to sizzling simply by following an easy-to-use system.

Living the Optimized Life is available to all of us, once we crack the code. Once you figure out all the pieces of the puzzle, your life can be a sizzling experience one crowded with success after success.

What Does Optimized Living Mean To You?

By adopting the Optimized Living system, you can create the world you've always dreamed of. What is it that you desire? A happy family life? A fulfilling career? Finally meeting those personal goals you set for yourself so many years ago?

The truth of the matter is that Optimized Living means something unique to each and every one of us. To some, it may mean spending more time with family. To others it may mean finally writing The Great American Novel. Or perhaps going back to school to completing a degree.

But Optimized Living – at its broadest – means enjoying a life unbridled by limits. It means desiring something, working for it and actually achieving it. Optimized Living means living and truly enjoying each day to its fullest.

Yes, that is a tall order. But it's not an impossible task. And I should know. Because I didn't always life the Optimized Life which I'm experiencing right now. At one time I felt trapped in a job I didn't enjoy and quite frankly wasn't very good at. I was in a marriage that was less than satisfying – both my spouse and myself. And even though I had great children, I didn't recognize the true extent of their greatness.

Then one day, I decided life had to change. There had to be more to living than what I saw or felt. So I began a total extreme makeover. Granted, my process at first was hit or miss, trial and error. But eventually I saw progress. I began to take pride in my job. I worked harder and eventually got a promotion, which paid more. And I was able to improve my family's standard of living.

Not only that, but my spouse and I are enjoying some of the best moments of our marriage. And our children? Well, I told you they were always great. But now I truly see just how magnificent they are.

Instead of waking up every day wondering what "bad" things could possibly befall me, I wake up envisioning all the amazing events that will take place as the day unfolds. My life has truly gone from so-so to sizzle.

This amazing change in both my actions and personality didn't go unnoticed by family and friends. Soon I had people asking me for my "secrets to life." They wanted to know how I made such a stunning transformation in such a short time.

Soon, I heard myself laying out the plan I used. Then it hit me. If so many of my friends felt this way, there must be others like me who also feel the same way. People who want desperately to turn their lives around but don't know where to start. That's when I decided that I need to write down everything I learned.

Simple Changes Bring Big Rewards

The changes I implemented in my life were simple. But searching them out and gathering them together was not so simple. In effect, I've already done the hard part. I've pieced together an outline and distilled it into a simple-to-understand, even simpler-to-follow set of instructions of living the Optimized Life.

Think about your life five, even ten years from now. Do you want to be at the same point then that you are now? Do you want to be merely surviving for the next decade or decade and a half?

There's a good chance that's exactly where you will be unless you learn the secrets to Optimized Living. They're easy to learn and even easier to use. And once you have these ideas and concepts, you'll never have to return to living a so-so life again.

Isn't it about time you experience a sizzling life? Isn't it about time you experience the true potential of what you can do? This is not dreaming, it's not some pie-in-the-sky unreachable goal.

Optimized Living is something everyone can achieve. Hey, I achieved it! And you can too!

An important step in the Optimized Living program is keeping your body healthy or healing your body from any damage already done to it. That's the premise of this book. It's difficult to feel good about your present and your future when you're not feeling your best. Enthusiasm takes energy (trust me, I know!) and energy is best obtained not through caffeine or supplements, but through foods. Superfoods, specifically.

Are you ready to take the next step to Optimized Living? Start preparing your body TODAY so you can enjoy the very best of everything. You know you deserve it. Now, it's your turn to experience Optimized Living!

Chapter 1: What Are Superfoods?

Discover how to transform your thinking, and indeed your life, from so-so to sizzling with the addition of these breakthrough, all-natural foods.

Start your Optimized Living program by giving your brain and your body every opportunity to perform at their most efficient, healthiest level ever. Let's face it. It's difficult to think clearly – let alone optimally – when your brain is filled with cobwebs for lack of oxygen, overwhelming stress or lingering toxins.

Additionally, how can you even begin to perform at your best when your thoughts are focused on worries about your health or even worse, you're focusing on the pain you may be experiencing from any number of diseases or disorders?

If you're really serious about morphing your life from so-so to sizzling through Optimized Living, you shouldn't neglect your nutritional needs. One of the quickest, safest and most natural ways to boost not only your thinking but your overall wellbeing is through diet. And superfoods are the quickest route you can take!

What Are Superfoods?

Superfoods are extraordinarily packed with vitamins, minerals, phytonutrients, bioflavoids, antioxidants and any number of other much-needed nutrients for optimal performance and thinking.

The prestigious Mayo Clinic calls this exciting newly emerging class as encompassing "the top health foods." In addition to all the nutrients, they're "solid sources" of much-needed dietary fiber.

But more than that, they're "nutrient dense," explains the Mayo Clinic, but not high caloric. That's good news for you. Between the fiber and the low calorie content, you can eat more of these foods than you can imagine without consuming an abundance of calories.

They've acquired a well-deserved reputation for not only providing you with vitality, turbocharged energy, robust health, but an oxygenated, well-nourished brain that responds quickly to the Optimized Living system. They're considered whole foods as opposed to processed or packaged foods.

In a nutshell, superfoods' abilities are two-fold. They simultaneously increase your nutritional profile, enhancing your physical health and longevity while helping to reduce your risk of developing many degenerative diseases.

The latest research credits this class of whole foods with an amazingly wide range of benefits from reducing your risk of developing cancer to aiding in the prevention of Alzheimer's Disease. Between those two, plug in this list of disorders that controlled scientific studies show may be alleviated or eliminated simply by reaching for Superfoods instead of sugary, starchy alternatives:

- Arthritis
- Depression
- Diabetes
- Hardening of the Arteries
- High Blood Pressure
- High Cholesterol
- High Triglycerides
- And much more!

Are you ready to discover what your new Optimized Living Diet should include? It's easiest to understand when you divide these foods into five broad categories. They include green, fruit and nut, herb, seaweed, and bee.

Natural Green Superfoods

The natural items found in the green category are, as you might expect, green leafy vegetables. We all know the tremendous benefits associated with them. Vegetables like kale, watercress, parsley, lettuce and endive, to name just a few, are the unsung heroes of the superfood green class.

Other great sources include broccoli sprouts, dandelion greens, chicory and mustard sprouts.

They're highly nutritious – everything a superfood should be – and readily available. Even with this, few of us eat as much of these as we should.

But there are so many more foods for you to choose from. Wheat grass falls into this class. This is the sprouted grass of wheat seed. And yes it's vastly different from whole grain.

Barley grass is another choice you have. Before skipping over this superfood, consider the following statistics. Barley grass contains eleven times more calcium than cow's milk, seven times more vitamin C and bioflavonoids than orange juice and five times more iron than spinach. If that doesn't qualify as a superfood, nothing does!

Wild blue-green alga is composed of 60 percent protein and an amazing complement of amino acids – even more than beef or soy beans. But more than that, it's also one of the best sources of beta carotene, the precursor to vitamin A as well as B vitamins and chlorophyll.

If you're really looking to improve your brain function and memory, this is the food you want to include in your Optimized Living Through Superfoods Diet.

Have you ever heard of spirulina? This is a cultivated micro-alga, eaten for thousands of years by the original cultures of both Mexico and Africa. With more than 70 percent protein content, it's one of the most abundant sources of protein known to mankind. Steak, in contrast, contains only 25 percent protein.

Chlorella is another alga – a fresh-water one – and also contains a complete protein profile, all the B vitamins as well as vitamin C and E. It also possesses a host of minerals that are just too numerous to list. If you're trying to prevent or relieve yourself of hardening of the arteries to help facilitate your Optimized Living, then this is a food you need to consider including in your diet.

Fruits and Nuts: Awesomely Powerful

What makes fruits and nuts an awesome staple of your Optimized Living Through Superfoods Diet? Antioxidants. These are substances that fight the natural accumulation of free radicals in your body. Free radicals are created as a natural consequence of your metabolism. But when your body begins to build up an excess of these – through exposure to pollution, cigarette smoking, exposure to radiation or the consumption of deep-fried foods – it can trigger any number of degenerative diseases.

Antioxidants are the superheroes of your body, sweeping the free radical villains away!

Berries of all kinds are being touted – and rightly so – as the most amazingly effective antioxidants Mother Nature ever made. But fruits of all kinds can help your overall health and especially nourish your brain.

Some of the lesser known of these fruits and berries include:

- Acai
- Coconuts
- Coconut Oil
- Goji berries
- Maca

- Noni
- Raw cacao

Perhaps You've Never Thought Of Herbs As Superfoods

Herbs are seldom the top choices of many individuals when it comes to superfoods. But this is one awesome category of nutrition. Herbs avail your body to a wide range of nutrients in a combination your body may not be receiving from other foods.

What are some of the best of the best you may want to fortify your diet with? Try any of these below. Just remember this is only a small portion of what's available to you.

- Aloe Vera
- Echinacea
- Ginseng
- Nettle

Of course, the easiest way to consume these is through supplementation. But this isn't necessarily the most advantageous to your body. It's better to use them in their whole form to get the most nutritious bang for your buck.

Seaweed? Really?

Okay, so seaweed perhaps doesn't sound extremely appetizing, but you'd be surprised. You'll also be amazed at all the health benefits you'll derive from these. They can help protect you – and your brain – from many of the toxic elements that are found everyone these days. The worst of these toxic offenders include heavy metal, pollutants, as well as radiation.

An added bonus of this superfood category is its incredible effectiveness at promoting weight loss. Each of these foods contains a naturally high percent of iodine which stimulates your thyroid gland, which in turn speeds up your metabolism. And, you know what happens from there!

Here are just a few of the choices you have when it comes to seaweed superfoods:

- Arame
- Dulse
- Kelp
- Kombu
- Nori
- Wakame

The Healing Power of Bees

The final category of superfoods which you may want to add to your Optimized Living Diet comes from the bees. Surprised? You shouldn't be. Bee pollen has long been held as a legendary nutritional supplement, supplying your body with energy.

In addition to bee pollen, though, you need to give propolis a try. This is the substance that coats the walls of bee hives, which many apiary keepers call the "most antiseptic place" in nature. Propolis has near-miraculous antibiotic effects. But more than that, it also has the ability to attack viruses and win – something antibiotics just can't do.

While you're checking out bee products, be sure to investigate royal jelly. It's been called a "powerhouse" of nutrients. In fact, it's the sole food the queen bee eats. She lives 40 times longer than the other hive members.

Armed with a working knowledge of superfoods and their astonishing health benefits, it's time to investigate a little closer how eating can possibly improve your thought process. Follow me to the next chapter to gain a fuller understanding of the relationship between nutrition and brain functions.

Chapter 2: TurboCharge Your Brain Power

Some 100 billion brain cells crave nourishment in order to operate at peak, optimized efficiency. Discover why the brain demands so much food and why Superfoods satisfy this need.

Your brain is a phenomenal organ. It's nothing if not dynamic, responsive and extremely efficient. It's very much a living, growing organ, creating new connections, developing more complex brain cells on demand. And in order to perform all these incredible functions it must be fueled by food.

It's important then that you know how the brain works and the nutrients needed in order for it to run at an optimized level.

You need to know your brain doesn't look exactly like you've probably been taught to visualize it. Remember those high school years, where a model of the human brain would sit in your biology class staring at you? It was probably pink and rubbery. Well, your brain is called "gray matter" for a reason. It really is gray.

About the size of your two fists placed together,

the brain is a very soft, almost pudding-like consistency packed with some 100 billion (that's billion with a "b") cells, called neurons. These neurons fuel our thinking, learning, feeling and yes, even our states of being.

Now, with that unbelievably large quantity of cells, you can imagine that nourishing this organ is imperative. As you may have guessed, the brain has a voracious appetite. Your brain craves good fats, proteins, and complex carbohydrates. Additionally, it hungers for vitamins, minerals, and phytonutrients. And then it's a thirsty organ – it requires plenty of water.

The neurons have been compared in shape to an outstretched hand, with the palm of the hand being the body and the tips of the fingers representing the dendrites and the rest of the fingers the axons.

The dendrites are crucial for the exchange of information and communications among the cells. The dendrites of one neuron receive the information from those of others. From there, the information is then passed through the axon to the body of the cell. The critical passing or delivery of the knowledge or information is called a synapse.

When your brain is gathering and passing

knowledge, more dendrites grow in response to this increased traffic. But the opposite can also occur. If your brain isn't acquiring and delivering new stimuli, then the dendrites are "pruned." They simply wither away from lack of use. The adage, "use it or lose it" has never been more applicable.

At one time it was thought that new dendrites couldn't be created once an individual had reached a certain stage of adulthood. At that point, the dendrites merely died off. This led to the belief that as people age, their brain power naturally declined. Now research shows this just isn't at all correct. Individuals well into their 50s, 60s, 70s and beyond can grow new dendrites with active use of the brain.

The Language of the Brain: Neurotransmitters

This information passed from neuron to neuron is coded in a specific language that each cell can comprehend, called neurotransmitters. These bits of knowledge are not only passed around, but are actually created in the brain itself. Specifically, they're made in the body of the neuron.

For the optimum and fastest creation as well as efficient delivery, your brain (once again) relies on the foods you feed it. This action needs proteins, vitamins and minerals. These hungry neurotransmitters are also rather delicate in their own way. They're susceptible to damage from the environmental toxins that enter our system. They are also harmed by "in-house" toxins, those which our bodies form as a natural part of living.

Your brain lives or dies, literally, depending not only on how much you use it, but on how you feed it. That's why superfoods are so very important in turbocharging your brain power.

But what kind of diet would help your brain work at its very best? This organ needs five fundamental classes of food in order to help you experience optimized living.

Good Fats

This should come as no surprise. After all, your brain is composed of 60 percent fat. Most of this fat is considered polyunsaturated. It aids in the maintenance of the flexible membranes of the cells in order to carry out the crucial constant communications. Not only that, but the fats are also instrumental in energy production and water storage.

The fats your brain craves most are omega-3 fatty acids whose sources include fish, nuts, seed and dark, leafy vegetables. You can also obtain omega-3 from corn, safflower and borage oil.

Not only does your brain crave good fats, but it's a battleground for position among the various types of fat you give your body. It's true! The other, less healthy fats, saturated and transfats actually displace polyunsaturated from your brain cells. So, it's not only important to eat foods high in omega-3 fatty acids, but it's imperative to eat as few of the other fats as well.

When these so-called bad fats predominate, your cells lose the physical flexibility they need for proper and swift communication. Just as these types of fats can produce sludge and crud in your arteries which block the efficient flow of oxygen, they do the very same thing in your brain. They reduce the oxygen supply which in turn also reduces the flow of the toxic waste of your brain.

Consider the results of the following research conducted on mice by Ann-Charlotte Granholm of the medical University of South Carolina, Charleston. She studied these animals on a diet which consisted mostly of polyunsaturated fats and a group which ate mostly trans- and saturated fats.

The animals were required to remember the hidden platforms of a maze. Those mice which had the "bad fats" diet learned at a slower rate than the members of the other group and made more errors. In fact, they performed approximately five times worse than those receiving a polyunsaturated diet.

Proteins

Your brain needs protein to build the neurotransmitters as well as create a support structure for the neurons. Specifically, protein provides your body with amino acids essential in these tasks.

Not only that, but certain proteins play important roles in your emotions and feelings. Tryptophan, for example, found in turkey and milk, is needed for the production of serotonin. This substance gives you that feeling of well-being.

Additionally, the amino acid tyrosine, found in almonds, avocados, bananas and meat, is responsible for the welling up of feelings of enthusiasm inside you. Pretty cool, huh?

But more than that, your brain uses these amino acids and restructures them, creating powerful antioxidants which help to protect your cells from damage due to toxic waste. Proteins also are vital for cell communication.

It's best to receive your protein from healthy

foods. Proteins aren't consumed in isolation. You can choose your chicken – the protein – either baked or fried. If your choice is fried, then you may also be feeding your brain unhealthy amounts of saturated or transfats.

The same goes for your choice of nuts. Don't think for a minute that honey roasted peanuts give you the same health benefits as those without that tasty topping. Carefully choose your protein sources. Ensure that they're part of healthy foods.

Carbohydrates

Okay. Let's get one thing straight here. We're not talking about simple, refined carbohydrates. Not soda. Not refined sugar. And definitely not all those packaged and provocative junk foods. Those items contribute to brain sludge the slowing of your thinking process. But it is true that your brain needs carbohydrates. They're its main energy source.

We're talking complex carbohydrates which your body, slowly, deliberately can then convert into sugar – or glucose – at a steady and healthy rate. Whole grain products are the foods of choice here. They not only contain the complex sugars your brain needs for energy, but they also possess fiber – a type of carbohydrate – which is responsible for slowing the absorption of the sugar.

Fruits and vegetables that are also great sources of complex carbohydrates include beans, brown rice, barley, oat bran, potatoes, oatmeal, oat bran, and yams.

Micronutrients

Micronutrients are aptly named. Your body and your brain really only need them in small amounts. But these small amounts make a big difference in your health – especially your brain health. Perhaps the most vital of these are the B vitamins. Not only do they produce much-needed energy for your brain cells, but they aid in the manufacture of specific neurotransmitters.

The B vitamins, for example, are essential to the production of serotonin that provides you with the all-important sense of well-being. These vitamins are also indispensable to the production of a substance best known by its initials, GABA, essential to focus and concentration.

Zinc is another micronutrient your brain craves, even though it may only use small amounts of it. This trace mineral is needed for the healthy growth of dendrites. It's also used in the repair of neurons.

But perhaps Zinc's most interesting task is in contributing to the "cementing" of new connections among the neurons. It is very much a needed nutrient in the formation of memory. If you were to examine the composition of your brain's hippocampus, the area responsible for both long- and short-term memory, you'd discover an inordinate amount of zinc.

Good superfood choices when it comes to this mineral include seeds and nuts, as well as healthy and properly prepared meats.

Calcium is another micronutrient more often associated with strong bones. But it's also used by your brain to maintain the electrical connection among the synapses. Not only that, but it contributes to the cleansing of your brain by either binding with or dislodging certain toxins.

Phytonutrients fall under this category as well. These are plant compounds that are immensely beneficial to your brain. While they don't actually help produce the neurotransmitters, they are indispensable to the repair as well as the protection of the neurons. They, in effect, act as antioxidants which neutralize the free radicals. In this way, phytonutrients actually help to protect your memory.

All of these micronutrients can be found in abundance in fruits and vegetables. Especially in the brightly colored ones.

Water

Six to eight glasses a day. We've all heard that. Maybe you've been one of those who question that rule of thumb. "Why does my body need that much water in a day?" you may ask. This becomes an especially difficult health rule to follow when your body isn't telling you that you're thirsty.

"If I needed water," you say, "my body would let me know."

The truth of the matter is that your body is in need of water for many reasons and it needs it in a quantity that we're not always aware. Your kidneys need the water to help prevent the formation of kidney stones.

Your brain needs this water because the neurons actually store water in the cells themselves. They're tucked away in balloon-like structures called vacuoles. These little reservoirs of water perform quite a few useful tasks. They maintain the tone of the membranes which in turn aid in the process of normal neurotransmission. Water plays a role in sweeping toxins from your brain and it prevents your brain from overheating. Should your brain overheat, it could result in a serious decline in thought processes and even brain damage.

In fact, according to Philippa Norman, MD, MPH, if you wait to drink until you're thirsty, your body is already experiencing dehydration. Normally, when you're "ready" to drink, your body has already lost two percent of its weight as well as a ten percent decline in your cognitive functioning.

10 Superfoods for Your Brain

1. Brazil Nuts

Rich in monounsaturated fats and a healthy dose of magnesium, Brazil nuts, according to Dr. Mehmet Oz, a medical expert and television host, aids the communication process between your body and brain.

2. Avocado

Rich in the essential healthy fats, eat this delicious superfood to ensure the efficient flow of blood to and through your brain.

3. Blueberries

Receive your antioxidants by eating blueberries. It's a natural "anti-aging" superfood for the brain. This berry contains an abundance of zinc, potassium, vitamins A, C and E.

4. Cold-water Fish

Reach for salmon among other cold-water fish. These are your best sources of omega-3 fatty acids. And we already know omega-3 is as good as it gets when it comes to natural fats. Indulge and enjoy!

5. Broccoli

It's rich in vitamin B6, as well as the antioxidant vitamin C. In addition, broccolis is a good source of calcium and folate, another member of the B vitamin group.

6. Baked Potato

Your brain loves the antioxidants in this food which flush out toxins. It's also grateful for the B6 and folate content which gives it the energy it needs.

7. Honey

Yes! Research reveals that this sweet natural nectar not only lessens the feeling of anxiety but it can boost your memory. It's especially effective at doing this in the aging brain.

8. Beans

Beans are great stabilizers of glucose. This makes them the perfect fuel food. Need brain energy? Reach for black beans, kidney beans or even lentils.

9. Dark Chocolate

Sometimes it does turn out that life is fair. The fact that a food so satisfying and delicious contains powerful antioxidants plus stimulants to boost concentration is proof of that. Dark chocolate also increases the production of endorphins, those wonderful neurotransmitters that kick start a good mood.

10. Coffee

Coffee? Yes. Believe it or not, the caffeine in this traditional beverage protects your brain from damage and helps to flush out toxins.

Superfoods for your brain are indeed an essential

aspect of your new Optimized Living Program. But these various foods are important in so many other ways as well to keep you healthy and ready to perform at your best.

In the next chapter we talk of how these powerful foods can create an optimized immune system which helps to guard against colds, flu, viruses and a host of other potential health problems. You can't do your best if you're not feeling your best.

Chapter 3: The Care and Feeding of Your Immune System

It's difficult to have an "Ah! Ha!" moment when your days are filled with "Ah! Choo!" moments. Discover why boosting your immune system may be the most underrated but most important secret to living the Optimized Life.

"Ah! Choo!"

We've all been through this scenario. Things are rolling right along in our lives, building a momentum in our career or at home or even in pursuing one of the Big Dreams of our life. Then a major cold hits you – or the flu. It could even be a seasonal outbreak of allergies that interrupts that momentum.

Why do I mention this? Because it's impossible to experience Optimized Living when you're busy battling a viral infection, fending off germs or lying in bed with the flu. Then there are those of us who are plagued by either seasonal allergies or chronic sinus problems.

In order to experience true Optimized Living, not only does your brain need to be operating at peak performance, but your body also needs to be working perfectly for you. You need to eliminate those "Ah! Choo!" moments so you can experience more "Ah! Ha!" moments.

I can hear you now. "I'm just prone to colds," you say. "I'm plagued with chronic sinus problems. There's nothing I can do about it."

What if I told you there IS something you can do about the frequency with which you develop colds? What if I told you there IS something you can do to help strengthen your body so it's more resistant to allergies, sinus disorders . . . and even more serious health challenges?

Yes, through providing your body with the nutrients it craves not only to stave off such challenges, but to live at an excitingly health level you might never have experienced before. The key to this incredible new path is in strengthening your immune system. . . fortifying your natural defense mechanism: your immune system.

What is the Immune System?

We all know we have an immune system, but few of us really understand how it works. Before we talk about what superfoods will turn your body into a fortress against germs, let's examine how the immune system works – briefly, of course.

The task of your immune system is to attack organisms and other foreign invaders that enter your body with the "intent" to cause disorder and disease. The system immediately runs through a series of steps which the medical community calls the immune response.

This system is composed of a close-knit network of cells, tissue and organs, all working as a team to keep you healthy. White blood cells, called leukocytes, are deeply involved in this work.

These leukocytes are classified in two broad categories: Phagocytes and lymphocytes. The phagocytes are those cells that actually "chew' the invading foreign substances. The lymphocytes don't destroy the invaders, but are rather the memory keepers of the system. They remember these foreign bodies in order to help your body destroy them.

They're the parts working when you get a flu shot. By injecting your system with a small amount of the flu virus itself, your immune system can then recall what these invaders look like, so to speak, and build a defense mechanism against them. The next time this virus enters your system, your immunity will be ready to deal with it effectively.

This is also the reason why, if you've already had

the chickenpox for example as a child, you never have to worry (typically, at least!) about contracting it again.

Three Types of Immunity

Sounds pretty cool, doesn't it? But that's not really the entire story. Your body actually has three separate types of immunity: innate, adaptive and passive. Which one kicks in to help provide us with Optimized Living depends, of course, on what situation we're facing.

Innate immunity, as you might guess, is the natural immunity you're born with. This is a generalized type of protection. You innate immunity is the reason you can be exposed to quite few germs on a daily basis without contracting diseases or falling ill.

Included in this category are what science calls external barriers to the body, specifically your skin and mucous membranes lining the nose, throat and other areas. These are, without a doubt, your body's first line of defense from those hoards of foreign invaders. This is also why any cut in your skin can expose you to infection. It's literally an opening to allow the invading germs entrance.

The second type of immunity is referred to as

adaptive. Sometimes you'll hear it called active. This type of protection develops and grows on a daily basis. When you're exposed to a germ your body has never encountered before it works to form an effective response. The adaptive immune system is the mechanism by which vaccinations work.

Finally, the third type is called passive immunity. This means that the immunity itself is actually borrowed from another source. Because of this, it only works for a short time at protecting your system. A classic example of this is an infant's natural immunity when being fed her mother's milk. Through the milk, the infant is actually receiving protection from the diseases her mother has already been exposed to.

An Aging Immune System

As you age, your immune system becomes less effective. This means, in turn, that you're more prone to acquiring colds, flu and other potentially damaging invaders. And you'd be surprised that you don't really need to be that old to experience an aging immune system. Research now reveals that your immune system (and alas, mine as well!) begins the imperceptible decline between the ages of 35 to 40!

Yikes! Yes, you have every right to be alarmed at

that news. And you'd be right to start trying to devise a way to mitigate or lessen that decrease in effectiveness as much as possible.

We've already established that you can't live the optimized life while you're battling or even worrying about what germs and other foreign invaders are preparing to ambush your health.

Sure, you could pump yourself full of all the vitamins your body needs to maintain this guard system by gulping down a handful of vitamins daily. This might become a tad tedious, though. Your immune system uses nearly the entire spectrum of nutrients. It uses vitamins A, B6, B12, C, D, and E.

But that's not the only building blocks it needs. It also requires a regular, steady supply of copper, folic acid, iron, selenium and zinc. You can see how you could spend your entire day taking this and that supplement and still not provide your body with the food it needs to effectively ward off diseases.

A much better method of nourishing your immune system is through . . . yep, you guessed it . . . superfoods. The only way to ensure that you're leading the Optimized Life you deserve is by ensuring your immune system is performing at it optimal.

Superfoods: Superheroes For Your Immunity

More effective than supplements! Able to heal your body faster than a speeding locomotive! Look! It's a food! It's a medicine! No, it's a superfood.

Indeed here is a list of the top 10 superfoods – and one "super-duper" bonus food – to build optimized immunity which gives you the ability to live an optimized life.

1. Beans

Again, beans make the top superfoods list. It's not only good for your brain, as we've already seen, but it's beneficial to your immunity as well. And again, you can thank its extraordinary antioxidant content.

Pick a bean. Any bean. Each offers you nothing but superfood nutrition. Green soybeans and soy are abundant sources of vitamin C, calcium, selenium and zinc. If you prefer, go for lentils and black-eyed peas. These have a tremendous amount of folate and zinc. Black and kidney beans are also a great source of folate.

2. Berries: Both Blue and Red

That's right! Reach for the berry of your choice the next time you're at the grocery store. Or reach for a variety of colors, because there's no wrong choice here. We've already been introduced to blueberries awesome ability to supply your brain with all the proper nutrients for optimized living.

But berries are also extremely useful to your immune system. Blueberries contain natural phytonutrients that protect your cells from getting damaged. At the same time, these nutrients also decrease inflammation, a contributing cause of pain and a precursor to a host of degenerative diseases.

Red berries – especially strawberries and raspberries – possess a phytochemical known as ellagic acid. Researchers believe this may help protect your body from carcinogens, those insidious foreign invaders waiting to ambush your good cells and spread cancer.

3. Fish

When it comes to bolstering your immune system, go fish! While just about any type of fish is a great immune builder, you need to steer clear of all fish that's fried. Some of the best sources of omega-3 fatty acids to be hauled out of the water include salmon, sardines, oysters, mackerel, tuna, rainbow trout, shark and herring.

Omega 3, by the way, is an anti-inflammatory substance. It reduces the inflammation throughout your body that may contribute to such degenerative diseases like cancer.

4. Whole Grains

With all the buzz about high-protein, low-carbohydrate diets, grains – even whole grains – have taken a hit lately. The truth is they keep showing up on every major list of superfoods. Do your immune system a favor by including these in your Optimized Living Program.

If you've avoided bread of any kind lately, it's time to bring it back. And if you've been eating white refined breads until now, it's time to toss these and replace them with the whole grain version. Your immune system will benefit greatly. Make the change a clean sweep, in fact. Instead of white rice, eat brown or wild rice. Eat corn tortillas instead of flour tortillas.

Surprisingly, it really doesn't take much to activate their health benefits. One serving a day. Yes, indeed! That's what the latest research shows. One serving of whole grains daily can lower your risk of heart disease and stroke.

This spectacular superfood is rich in zinc and selenium – just what your immune system ordered! Plus, it also has a host of phytonutrients that can protect you from cancer.

5. Good Grape!

Now, here's some "grape" news. This tasty, unassuming fruit can be your ticket to super perfect immunity. This is especially true if you choose the dark-colored grapes: red, purple and blue. These babies are jam packed with phytonutrients and antioxidants that are widely believed to supercharge your immune system from even such serious diseases as cancer and heart disease.

Specifically, two of these phytochemicals, anthocyanin and proanthocyanin, target your immune system. Grapes are also rich in vitamin C and selenium – two more nutrients your body's defense mechanisms needs.

6. Green Leafy Vegetables

The greener the better. Make this your mantra if you're searching for the best fortification for your immune system. When you think green, think kale, collard greens and spinach, just for starters. But don't stop there – expand your green horizons. If you've never tried Asian greens, now's a good time to taste them.

Check out the taste of rocket and sliver beet as well. By the way, now is the perfect time to take that decorative sprig of parsley off your plate and munch it down.

What makes dark green vegetables so powerful? Wow! Just about everything. Let's start with the familiar basic vitamin line-up: A, C, and E. Add calcium, magnesium and potassium to that profile. And we're not even talking about the amazing antioxidant phytonutrient kaempferol. This substance may have cancer-fighting properties, according to the latest research.

Green leafy vegetables. Need we say more?

7. Orange Vegetables

If you're going the full spectrum of colors, then be sure to include carrots, white butternut squash and acorn squash. These are all classified as orange vegetables. While not particularly a scientifically derived division, it's useful when you shop. In addition to an incredible variety of phytonutrients, these foods also contain the old standbys for your immune system – vitamins C and A.

8. Go Nuts Over Nuts!

Go ahead! It really is okay. Well, it's more than okay. Nuts have long held the reputation as being high in fat and even higher in calories. In a nutshell, everything we were told to avoid. Now we understand that nuts of all kinds -- from almonds to Brazil nuts and pistachios – are filled with good fats.

Not only that but they just may be nature's most balanced food. In addition to these wonderfully healing fats, nuts also have just the right amount of protein and carbohydrates. The nut containing the greatest quantity of omega-3 fatty acids is the walnut. The white Brazil nut has the most selenium content of all nuts.

9. Sweet Potatoes

Think white potatoes only even more nutritious. These tubers are finally coming into their own. If your family was like mine when I was growing up, we only ate sweet potatoes once a year: Thanksgiving.

But all that is changing now – and changing rather fast. Sweet potatoes offer your immune system with vitamin C and B6 as well as potassium, calcium and fiber. And they are an astonishingly abundant source of vitamin A.

Sweet potatoes. Not just for holidays anymore!

10. Tea

Green. Black. It makes little difference. Now research shows that all tea is a blessing to your immunity. Tea contains the same two phytochemicals found in red berries – anthocyanin and proanthocyanin, known as inflammation fighters. Additionally, tea also contains an antioxidant called catechin, which the medical community thinks prevents potential damage from cancer cells.

Bonus Superfood

That's the top 10 list of immune-building superfoods. But there's one we haven't mentioned because it stands heads and shoulders above all the others. That, at least, is the professional opinion of Chris Kresser, author of the highly popular and very informative Healthy Skeptic blog and a licensed acupuncturist.

What food is it? Many of you aren't going to like the answer.

Beef liver.

Some of you, however, are jumpy around singing, "I told you so! I told you so!"

Okay, so it's not just beef liver that's of tremendous benefit to your immune system, though it's the crème de la crème of livers. It comes to the table with impeccable credentials:

- 6 times the iron content of kale
- 30 times the vitamin B6 content of ground beef
- Incredibly abundant in vitamin A
- Excellent source of folic acid
- Rich in zinc
- Packed with copper
- Great source of selenium

Not only is liver high in nutrients, Kresser explains, but it's low in price. On your next trip to the grocery store, take notice. You'll see exactly what he means.

For Optimized Living, you should eat three to four ounces of liver weekly.

There's a variety of superfoods listed here from which to choose to build an amazingly fortified immune system. And this can mean the difference between being plagued with colds all winter long, with the latest strain of the flu and other sinister health-stealing foreign invaders.

The next step in leading the Optimized Life: your weight. Don't groan. With your growing knowledge of superfoods combined with what you're about to learn, you'll discover that reaching your optimal weight in order to enjoy Optimized Living is much easier than it's ever been before.

Chapter 4: Superfoods and Weight Loss: The Golden Key to Optimized Living

Discover how you can truly optimize your life by losing weight through a superfoods eating plan. It's actually easier than you think.

The Standard American Diet is based on convenience. More of us than ever before are eating "fast foods." Who has time for a leisurely meal these days?

More of us visit the frozen food section of the grocery store. Frozen dinners are far less of a hassle than making a real meal.

And more of us than ever before are eating -- in large quantities -- foods that are boxed, canned and other pre-packaged and processed foods.

For far too many of us eating is merely another item on our "to do" list. Eat as quickly as possible – check it off as completed, and continue with our next item.

The Standard American Diet – aptly abbreviated SAD according to some nutritionists – is not based on nutrition. It will never be able to supply you with the nutrients you need to enjoy

Optimized Living.

In fact, the average American eats 31 percent more processed and packaged foods than fresh foods, according to The New York Times. While it makes your life easier, it certainly doesn't help you live longer. Studies show that diets with higher levels of fat, salt, and sugar only provide the general population with higher rates of heart disease, diabetes and obesity.

It's not a very beneficial way to eat if you want to experience Optimized Living. It takes little effort, if you really give it some thought, to reach for a superfood over a candy bar for a late afternoon snack.

Because you're serious about enjoying all the benefits of Optimized Living, you'll undoubtedly want to take advantage of these wonderfully nutritious and incredibly healthy foods that can help you shed your extra pounds.

And when you do, one of the many benefits will be more energy than you've ever imagined possible. Actually, the benefits of losing weight are quite amazing – especially when you accomplish this through the consumption of superfoods.

In addition to feeling more energetic and

reducing your risk for developing a myriad of degenerative diseases, here are just a few of the other rewards you'll reap:

- A better, deeper night's sleep
- Less aches and pains
- Lower cholesterol levels
- Reduce blood pressure levels
- Get you moving easier and faster
- Improved breathing
- Increased self-esteem
- Alleviate depression

Losing weight, according to a new study, actually improves your quality of life, placing you squarely on the road to Optimized Living. According to the results of research published in the American Journal of Preventive Medicine, Americans have lost twice the number of "quality-of-life" years due to obesity from 1993 to 2008 than previously.

Your goal is not only to maintain a high quality of life, but improve on that with Optimized Living. That can be done painlessly by indulging yourself with superfoods.

I hesitate even to call eating superfoods a diet. It really isn't. It's much more a change in lifestyle. In fact, merely lessening your dependency on fast foods, processed and prepackaged foods while increasing your consumption of superfoods will start you on the path to Optimized Living.

What Superfoods Are Most Suited to a Weight Loss Plan?

The truth of the matter is every superfood is an ideal weight loss food. So any food in this book can be eaten with the confidence that it will help you drop those extra pounds – whether you have five or ten to lose or 60 or 70 you want to shed.

But here are ten of the most basic. Start with these, add others as you're ready and you'll be increasing your energy and enjoying Optimized Living before you know it.

1. Apple

Either alphabetically or nutritionally classified, the apple tops every list of weight loss superfoods. And with good reason. One medium apple is the equivalent of one serving of fruit. Within this often under rated apple lies a hidden treasure of nutrition: four grams of soluble fiber, a mere 95 calories and 14 percent of your daily requirement of vitamin C.

Not only that, but because of its generous fiber content, eating an apple shortly before a meal can help you eat less.

2. Tomato

Low in calories, high in nutrition, the tomato is an excellent dieting choice. It's not only an abundant source of vitamin A and C, but is rich in the antioxidant lycopene as well. This relatively newly discovered antioxidant may provide you with added protection against heart disease and cancer as well as the eye disorder macular degeneration.

Unlike many antioxidants, lycopene is actually more powerful when it's cooked than raw. But in any form, the tomato is still one of the healthiest choices you can make. Here's a suggestion. Cut a tomato in half. Sprinkle parmesan over it, then place it in the broiler until the cheese melts. It makes the ideal superfoods snack.

3. Salmon

Yes, we already know fish is rich in omega-3 fatty acids which help provide you with the super nutrition you need to live the Optimized Life. But it also is rich a rich source of protein, calcium, and vitamins A and D.

Grill it. Sautee it. Bake it. Drizzle a little lemon juice over it and serve it with brown rice (another excellent superfood!). Now, you're eating a superfoods meal. Congratulations!

4. Green Tea

Tea is another superfood we're already familiar with. But it could be doubly effective for you when you're on a weight loss plan. That's because it's incredibly effective at raising your metabolism rate. Give it a try.

5. Broccoli

I know it seems to be the designated food people love to hate, but once you understand its health benefits, you may have second thoughts about this wonder food. It's loaded with fiber and the super nutrition of the vitamins A and C. In addition, it's rich in folate. On top of that, broccoli is a low-calorie food. One cup of chopped broccoli contains just 30 calories.

6. Banana

Don't be surprised this fruit is on the list of superfoods. And don't believe the voices that say the banana isn't good for you – because it just isn't so!

Yes, it may be a little starchier than other fruits, but in many ways it's one of the ideal super fruits for weight loss. A medium banana – because of its fiber content – can keep you full and satisfied for hours.

A banana contains potassium, which helps to keep your muscles strong and your nerves healthy. It also helps to lower your bad cholesterol. It's also a good source of vitamin C, and they deliver all this for only 130 calories. It really doesn't get much better than this.

7. Avocado

At one time considered a food off limits for dieters, you can now enjoy this scrumptious fruit. It contains a fatty acid known as oleic acid, which can actually stave off those hunger pangs. It's worth eating just for that! But your body will thank you for the protein and carbohydrates you'll be giving it, too!

8. Egg

Oh yes, the incredible, edible egg as the television commercial explains. Welcome back omelets and scrambled eggs. Go ahead, eat an omelet for breakfast and pack it with delicious superfoods of the vegetable variety – especially broccoli, peppers and onions.

Once thought to raise your cholesterol level, eggs in moderation are now considered a superfood. This compact food, with only 75 calories is packed with enough vitamins, minerals and other nutrients to make your head swim. They include:

- Calcium
- Magnesium
- Zinc
- Sodium
- Copper
- Manganese
- Phosphorus
- Selenium
- Potassium
- Thiamine
- Riboflavin
- Pantothenic Acid
- Niacin
- Folate
- Vitamin B12
- Vitamin B6
- Vitamin A
- Vitamin D
- Vitamin E
- Vitamin K

If you don't have time to eat breakfast, an omelet for dinner provides an interesting change of pace!

9. Almond Butter

If you like the amazing superfood almonds, then you'll love almond butter. It has what appears to be "magical" abilities to actually lower the glycemic index of bread. It's true. Researchers took a group of people and divided them into two groups. One group ate a plain slice of white bread – the highest food on the glycemic index. The other group ate white bread, but spread almond butter on it.

Those who ate only the bread experienced a large spike in their glucose levels – as you might well expect. Those who ate it with the almond butter experienced a much lower jump in their glucose measurement. The study was conducted at the University of Toronto.

10. Pomegranate

No, not the juice, though certainly it is a superfood in its own right. But in this case, munch on the pomegranate seeds themselves. These are loaded with antioxidants, fiber and folate. And they have the added benefit of taming your sweet tooth.

Don't know how to eat them? Put them in salads, especially those made with raw baby spinach. You'll love it. Guaranteed.

Dig into these superfoods. But don't limit yourself. Remember this is only the first step on your new path to Optimized Living. You'll learn exactly what we mean when we say living the Optimized Life when you lose weight and gain unbelievable amounts of energy. Your mind will also be clear because you won't fear the development of the many degenerative diseases that accompany being overweight.

As you lose that weight, you may want to investigate the next chapter. How you can eat your way – with superfoods, of course – to healthier, glowing skin.

Chapter 5: Superfoods and Healthy Skin

Meet your body's largest organ. While we've always been told that beauty is only skin deep, the health of your skin is, in reality, a reflection of your overall well-being. You're not experiencing Optimized Living if your skin is less than healthy. And here's why.

Beauty is only skin deep.

Here's one adage we need to toss – and the sooner the better.

Yes, there's no doubt you need glowing skin to be beautiful. But you'll never reach true healthy skin with make-up and other cosmetics alone. The truth of the matter is that the appearance of your skin is a bell weather for your overall health.

Did you know that the skin is your body's largest organ? Yes, it really is an organ, as essential to your continued good health as your heart, liver or kidneys.

If up until now you thought it is odd that a book on Optimized Living would talk about skin, you now understand why it is.

Meet Your Body's Largest Organ

Right about now, you may be wondering how the skin contributes to your super health. The top layer of your skin is called the epidermis. Its function is two-fold. First, it protects your system from foreign invaders. Any time you cut yourself or have any open wound you're also at a greater risk of acquiring an infection. And now the next time you do get a cut or a scrape, you'll see the importance of taking good care of it, no matter how small.

But the skin also acts as a "barrier" for unwanted toxins in your body. It releases poison which, if remained, would compromise your immune system. The skin, in effect, is more than just a "petty face" for us. It's a hard-working vital organ. It hydrates itself and renews itself in addition to protecting the rest of your body.

In addition to nourishing it with superfoods, you need to ensure your skin receives all the water it requires. And I don't mean through showering and bathing (although that's a great idea too!). You've always been told you should drink between six to eight glasses of water daily. This is just one of the reasons why you need to heed this advice.

Adequate water intake combined with plenty of fiber in your diet is the perfect prescription to flushing out toxins which may be blocking your ability to lead the Optimized Life.

Proper skin care, then, is one of the lesser known secrets to Optimized Living because beauty really isn't just skin deep. Keeping your skin healthy will not only keep your skin looking younger longer, but it'll keep your body performing at its peak.

The 10 Superfoods for Healthy, Vibrant Skin

The following are among the 10 best superfoods targeting skin health. If you include these in your new Superfoods for Optimized Living meal plans, you'll not only experience healthier, softer skin (with fewer wrinkles, by the way) but you'll be taking a giant step (which many individuals don't even know about) towards Optimized Health.

1. Turkey

The meat once reserved for only Thanksgiving and Christmas has emerged as a superfood – especially when we're talking healthy, glowing skin. The substances found in turkey play a vital role in reducing the deterioration of your collagen. Considering that 65 percent of your skin is made of collagen, and it's the main structural protein binding your skin together, delaying its demise can translate into younger looking skin.

Of course, organic turkey is your best choice. But if you can't locate any, then non-organic is better than none at all.

2. Bell Peppers

Take your pick, red or yellow. Or mix them together. In any case, your skin certainly is the beneficiary. Red and yellow peppers are an amazingly rich source of antioxidants. One half of a pepper contains 142 mg of vitamin C. That's more than twice your daily requirement and (now get this) only 20 calories.

What does this antioxidant content mean to you? It means extra protection from the sun, according to the latest research coming from the University of Arizona.

3. Olives

You probably never thought about olives as being nourishment for your skin, let alone a superfood. But listen to this. "The more olives you eat, the less wrinkled your skin appears."

That's the discovery from research performed at Monash University in Australia. Now that's some superfood for thought.

4. Olive Oil

How would you like to receive the benefits of olives without actually eating them? Olive oil is the perfect choice for anyone who doesn't care for the fruit of the olive tree. Actually this oil is already well known as a healthy choice. Because of its abundant omega-3 fatty acid content, some nutritionists say you should use at least one tablespoon daily. It's perfect to use with vinegar on salads. Your best bet is to start with the extra virgin variety. Not only is this variety cold pressed, which means that it retains its natural flavor, but it's free from chemical additives.

5. Watermelon

This luscious summertime fruit needs to be eaten all your round if you want to keep your skin healthy. It helps to hydrate your skin which is vital for that supple texture, but it helps you retain a soft complexion. Watermelon contains plenty of vitamin C, potassium, and lycopene. In addition, this is the ultimate superfood to eat for achieve the perfect delicate balance of water and nutrients.

6. Oysters

This seafood is legendary for its aphrodisiac qualities. But there's another reason you may want to eat them: to keep your skin glowing. They're a great source of zinc, which we already know contributes to skin healthy.

7. Egg Whites

Yes, I know we've already mentioned the incredible, edible egg as a superfood. But the white of the egg is a great source of nutrients in its own right. The whites are rich in the essential trace mineral zinc, necessary to firm, younger-looking skin.

8. Walnuts

Within this superfood, you can improve the quality of your skin by eating merely a handful a day. Walnuts have everything your skin craves, especially omega-3 fatty acids and vitamin E. They can be conveniently inserted into your meals by adding these nutty treats to salads, pasta and even dessert.

9. Kiwi

If you're looking for a delicious way to maintain vital-looking skin, eat this antioxidant-rich fruit.

The small but mighty kiwi is jam-packed with vitamin C. One medium kiwi has 74 mg of this outstanding nutrient and antioxidant and is only 45 calories.

10. Dark Chocolate

Yes, I saved the very best for last. All the chocoholics are now celebrating by breaking open a candy bar. And well, they should. Yes, isn't it good to know your skin loves dark chocolate as much as you do? It not only helps to hydrate your skin, but it also serves as a great protector from sun damage. Here's a hint when choosing your chocolate: make sure it contains a minimum of 60 percent cacao.

Now that you have a great start to Optimized Living through Superfoods, it's time to understand a little more about why proper nutrition is a vital part of your health. Specifically, it's time to learn a little more about antioxidants which in and of themselves can help you live free from the fear of many degenerative diseases. Now that's an Optimized Life!

Follow me to the next chapter to see how you can reduce your risk of developing such diseases as heart disease, arthritis, and even cancer just through smart food choices.

Chapter 6: The Amazing Power of Antioxidant Superfoods

You've heard about them. You've read about them. And you've probably been eating many of these superfoods already. Now learn how antioxidants work and how to rate them to truly experience Optimized Living.

It's enough to make your head spin. The unabridged explanation of how antioxidants perform their near miraculous healing powers. This amazing biological show has a large cast: atoms, protons, neutrons, free radicals. And that's only a portion of the stars of the show.

Oh, yes, they all give stellar performances. But for our purposes a quick explanation reveals enough to help you fully grasp the impact of the effects of antioxidants.

It's hard not to know that some of the important nutrients which are the stars of the antioxidant show include vitamins A, C, and E. Additionally, substances such as lycopene are also very effective in this role.

It's also hard not to know that antioxidants are reputed to be responsible for helping to reduce your chances of nearly every degenerative disease from arthritis to heart disease, diabetes and cancer.

A Quick Overview of How Antioxidants Work

Any detailed explanation of this process gets confusing. You can drown in a sea of technical terms trying to figure it all out. Nonetheless, it's important that you have a general idea of how these wonderful naturally occurring substances work.

Antioxidants actually attach themselves to the harmful substances within your body called free radicals. Free radicals are highly unstable byproducts formed through as a result of natural chemical reactions which take place continuously in your body.

Your system produces an inordinate amount of these when you're exposed to an excessive amount of environmental toxins. This could include items we all know aren't good for us, like cigarette smoke, ultraviolet radiation and air pollution.

The free radicals, if not scooped up by the antioxidants, attack your cells in their search for stability. It's the attack of the free radicals which, after a length of time, causes degenerative diseases.

Results of years of scientific study now have researchers believing that antioxidants work in two ways. First, they can neutralize and render impotent the free radicals before damage is caused. But, secondly, they also help to reduce existing damage. This makes them an especially attractive component of the Optimized Living system.

The ORAC Rating System for Antioxidants

If you're wondering if some antioxidants are more potent than others, the answer is a resounding, unqualified yes. Until recently, though, it proved difficult for you and I, as average consumers, to actually determine which superfoods were superior to others. (See, even all superfoods aren't created equal!)

We, in effect, had no method by which to judge an antioxidant's ability to fight free radicals. And we certainly had no idea how much of these antioxidants were in the foods we ate.

Enter ORAC. Everything has changed. This rating system has turned the nutritional community on its head. And, in the process, allows you to map out your eating plan to create your own personal Optimized Living through Superfoods meal plan.

ORAC stands for Oxygen Radical Absorption Capacity. This system measures the ability of foods to render useless the free radicals and remove them from your body. The theory behind this measurement is that the fewer free radicals, the lower your risk of developing degenerative diseases as well as a slowing of the aging process.

A score of 400 is good. Your average fruits and vegetables hover around this range. But in order to create an Optimized Life, then set your sites higher. The higher the ORAC rating the more potentially powerful the antioxidant superfood is. Finally, you can truly say you control your health.

Examples of foods with an average score are peas, carrots, corn and lettuce. Healthy foods within their own right – and certainly ones you should be including in your diet. But now take a look at the chart below. It documents twelve most antioxidant-rich superfoods currently known to science. (I say this because scientific research is constantly breaking new ground. Some researcher somewhere may be testing a food that will be on this list tomorrow!)

Once you look at this list, I guarantee you'll be running to the grocery store even before you finish reading this chapter.

The Top 12 List

Superfood	ORAC Rating
Cacao Powder, 1 Tablespoon	4017
Blueberries, ½ Cup	4848
Pomegranate, 1	4950
Black Plum, 1	5003
Pecans, one handful	5086
Cranberries, ½ cup	5271
Apple, 1	5609
Cinnamon, 1 teaspoon	6960
Artichoke, 1	11,000
Goji Berries, ½ cup	18,980
Acai Berries, ½ cup	74,780

The natural tendency, now that you're aware of the tremendous benefits of these superheroes, is to load up on these at the expense of other superfoods. While in theory that may be a reasonable idea, in actuality it's not. All superfoods offer a wide variety of benefits. Many of them have already been documented. But we have no idea what benefits the scientific community has yet to find.

Look at the tomato as just one example. While it's already been beneficial, it's now in the spotlight as a true superfood because of its lycopene content, an amazing warrior against cancer. And it didn't even make the top twelve list!

Simple Measure to Ensure Optimized Living Through Superfoods

If you want to truly experience Optimized Living, of course you're going to choose some of your superfoods from this ORAC rating. But there are also several other methods you must also incorporate into your dietary habits. Check these out below to achieve a true and satisfying Optimized Life.

Choose Variety

Don't restrict yourself to only a few foods – even those superheroes of superfoods with astounding ORAC ratings. By enlarging your range of options, you'll be receiving greater health benefits – sometimes in ways we don't fully understand yet.

Choose Fruits and Vegetables

As you've already seen, fruits and vegetables contain untold health benefits. You can't go wrong choosing these naturally wholesome, antioxidant-rich foods – even if they aren't on the top 12 list.

Choose Fiber

Fiber not only helps you feel fuller, which in turn helps with weight control, but it can help lower your risk of developing many degenerative diseases, those most associated with the aging process.

Choose Moderation

You can't go wrong when you select a variety of foods in moderate amounts. It only makes sense that your body demands diverse vitamins, minerals and phytonutrients. It's a wonderfully complex biological system you're carrying around with you. It needs a wonderfully healthful array of foods to keep it at its optimal level.

Choose to Lessen Your Dependence On Sugar

That's admittedly difficult. Your dependence on sugar grows the more you reach for sugar-laden cola, candy bars and other snack foods.

You'll discover exactly how dependent your body is on sugar as you wean yourself off of it.

Choose to Eat Fewer Fried Foods

We've known for years that fried foods, especially those fried with transfats, can slowly whittle away your good health. But eating these foods also creates an in balance in your body's omega-6 and omega-3 fats ratio. Both are certainly essential to health, but they must be kept in a delicate balance, or disease can strike.

Living the Optimized Life

By choosing high ORAC foods, eating a variety of fruits and vegetables as well as whole grains, you'll be supplying your system with the best nutrients possible. You'll be giving it nutrients we already know will go a long way to creating an Optimized Life. But, you'll be feeding it beneficial nutrients science has yet to discover. Talk about cutting-edge living.

There's one other way to turbocharge your health: combine certain superfoods to create a synergistic reaction. Follow me to the next chapter to see exactly how to increase your potential for Optimized Living exponentially.

Chapter 7: Synergized Superfoods Strategies

Discover how to add the oomph to an already energized superfoods eating plan simply by knowing what food combinations to eat. It's called synergy – and it can help you take that giant leap from living to Optimized Living.

Consider this the dynamic duo section of the book. Like superheroes Batman and Robin, pairing two superfoods can bring you even more nutritional benefits than either one eaten alone. This effect is called synergy. It's the result of the sum of two or more items which creates a larger, more spectacular outcome than either item can accomplish on its own.

Just which benefits you receive and how much they're enhanced depends on what foods you're actually eating and the specific results of these foods. Each combination offers a unique, healthy advance in gaining optimal health.

And it's the theme of this chapter. If you are excited about beginning the Optimized Living program… if you want to see results as quickly as possible... then you want to carefully read this chapter, re-read it – and then head straight for the grocery store. You'll want to take this quantum leap to Optimized Living as quickly as possible.

Below are seven of the most effective dynamic duos in the superfoods realm. Keep in mind, though, this is just a start as you progress on your journey to a more energized life.

1. Iron and Vitamin C

The first superhero pair we're examining is probably the most common: iron and vitamin C. The next time you order a breakfast, be sure to include orange juice when you eat your eggs and meat.

Vitamin C, best exemplified by orange juice, increases your body's absorption rate of iron. This is especially important when you eat plant-based foods. Your body is a little less efficient at using the iron it receives from vegetables than it is in using the iron found in meat. But if you eat or drink anything that possesses vitamin C, you create an astounding synergistic reaction. Your body, in effect, has the ability to absorb more of the iron.

If you're low in iron or feeling sluggish then don't pass on those potatoes with that breakfast, either. Potatoes are a good source of vitamin C. That means the effects of your eggs, bacon, sausage or ham – all iron-containing foods can actually be given a boost when you eat that side of potatoes. Who knew?

Think, also, of pairing kale and oranges. Or making a salad that includes spinach, definitely a food possesses iron, with tomatoes, yellow and red bell peppers and broccoli. Now you have more than just a delicious salad – you have a synergized effect occurring in your body! Doesn't it make a salad much more attractive and exciting alternative now?

Other foods known for their rich iron content include oatmeal, tofu, wheat germ, quinoa and starchy beans.

Among your choices in the vitamin C category are all citrus fruit, kiwi, guava, strawberries and Brussels sprouts and potatoes. To truly make this work for you, be sure to choose *your* favorite foods. In this way, the resulting synergism for which you're striving will fell much less obligatory and more like a feast!

2. Inulin and Calcium

Ever hear of inulin? It's a type of fiber that performs a most important balancing act. It keeps your intestinal good and bad bacteria from overwhelming each other. Inulin, not to be confused with the hormone insulin, has one other specific duty: it contributes to the strength of your bones.

Now you can understand why it synergizes with calcium in optimizing your bone density. Not sure what are good sources of inulin? Try such diverse foods as bananas, whole-wheat flour, asparagus, garlic, celery, chicory, onions, artichokes and dandelion greens.

Pair any of these with the following calcium-containing foods: cheese, yogurt, milk, broccoli, kale and canned salmon (be sure to buy the variety with the bones). Don't forget that sardines are also a great source of calcium as well as fortified orange juice, almonds, almond milk, soy and rice.

The next time you add bananas to your cereal, you're doing more than just enjoying a breakfast. You're moving quickly along the path of Optimized Living! Now doesn't that feel great?

3. Calcium and Vitamin D

Like love and marriage . . . or a horse and carriage . . . calcium and vitamin D are a natural synergistic pair. This particular vitamin needs to be present in order for your body to actually put the calcium to use. Otherwise, it's just a wasted trace mineral.

Think milk, here. It naturally contains calcium; then it's fortified with vitamin D. Perhaps someone knew something more than we did all along. If you're interested in other great combinations that can achieve this effect, try grilled salmon with sautéed kale, a broccoli and cheese omelet and a tuna melt on whole grain bread with low-fat cheese.

We've already reviewed some of the most common vitamin C-rich foods. Take those foods and eat them alongside these stars of the vitamin D world: salmon, sardines, egg yolks, fortified soy, rice and almond milk.

4. Vitamin E and Vitamin C

Are you looking to maintain good eyesight? Look no further than vitamin E. And it can stand alone and help you do this. But when you allow it to work with the amazingly versatile antioxidant, vitamin C, well . . . you can just guess that your body experiences benefits of exponential proportions. If you have ever eaten a salad with mandarin organs and almonds, then your system has experienced this superfood synergy.

Foods rich in vitamin E include: almonds, and almond butter, peanuts and peanut butter, wheat germ, sunflower seeds and soybeans.

5. Vitamin K and Good Fats

It's as simple as eating a salad with olive oil and vinegar. Really. It doesn't get much easier than that, now does it? You probably have eaten this thousands of times, but never realized how much your body truly benefited from it.

The essential pairing contained within this is the good fats working in the presence of vitamin K. And you know exactly what fats we're talking about – unsaturated fats. And we're specifically targeting those vital omega-3 fatty acids found in the oil and vitamin K found in those dark, green vegetables. Toss in almonds and you've added a little bit more of the unsaturated fats for good measure.

Unsaturated fatty acids are legendary for their ability to reduce your cholesterol level. And vitamin K is responsible for the proper clotting of your blood. But there's a secret that's seldom revealed. Vitamin K is actually useless unless it's accompanied by the good fats.

So where exactly can you find vitamin K? Look no further than kale, spinach, Swiss chard, Brussels sprouts, cabbage, broccoli and turnip greens.

Of course, the good fats are mostly found in cold-water fish, all oils like olive, canola and flaxseed are especially chocked full of the good fats. So are nuts of all kinds.

6. Sulphur Compounds and Zinc

Sulphur compounds, you wonder. Sure. You've probably eaten many foods containing these amazing substances and not even have known it. Well, you eat them if you like garlic and onions at least. These two pungent plants play an important role in increasing your body's natural ability to absorb zinc. And zinc, in turn, is vital to a healthy, strong and vigilant immune system. Eat these foods together and you can understand how it will supercharge your immune system.

Now you have a healthy reason – beyond personal tastes – to eat these rich superfoods with onions and garlic: whole grains, brown rice and legumes.

Adding onions to any sandwich made with whole wheat bread creates not just a dietary delight, but a dynamic duo synergized reaction.

7. Catechin and Vitamin C

If you recall from an earlier chapter, tea—either green or black – are considered superfoods because of they are a great source of catechin, a flavonoid especially effective at protecting you from developing a variety of serious health issues, most notably heart disease and cancer. Yeah, they're that important.

After your body digests the catechin in the tea, there's only approximately one fifth of the original content left that's actually available to your body for practical use. One way to increase this amount is by drinking tea along with vitamin C based foods.

And as you probably guessed, the easiest way to do this is through adding a lemon wedge to your drink. What does this small gesture do? Plenty. The presence of this amazingly versatile antioxidant increases the amount of catechin available for your body's use by an astounding 80 percent. Now, can you even think of drinking tea without lemon?

There are seven initial ways in which to take a quantum leap to Optimized Living using the synergistic strategy. As large a step this is, you're only just beginning your journey. Imagine how great you'll feel after you make these dynamic duos of superfoods your trusted protectors of your health!

Conclusion: The Start of a Brand-New You!

I always hate writing conclusions. They seem so, well, final. This is the part of the book I must say goodbye to you, at least temporarily. But it's not the end of your learning about Optimized Living. Nor is it the end of your superfoods journey.

In fact, your journey is just beginning. You're well on your way to a new, improved you. You're keeping the very essence of you are, but you're adding a new element: super health.

Imagine for a moment how much you can achieve when you feed your body the nutrition it craves. Imagine your brain on superfoods. Do me a favor. For a moment think about the goal you'd love to accomplish. Think of it regardless of whether you believe you can achieve it or not.

Got it pictured in your head. Good. You know what that means don't you? It means you can achieve it. Yes it does! Once you start using the Optimized Living system, you'll discover how easy it really is.

And you can start right now, by eating for Optimized Living. How could you ever hope to achieve that very important dream without preparing your body with super nutrition?

If you believe that the changes asked of you here are too large – and depending on your current diet, the ideas may seem overwhelming – then embrace the changes one at a time. No one said you had to throw all of the food out of your pantry. You certainly can add the most appetizing selections you've found in here.

As you continue along your Optimized Living journey, you'll be eager, even impatient, to add more antioxidant-rich, nutritionally abundant foods to your eating plans. Guaranteed!

And you'll discover how Optimized Living can morph your life from so-so to sizzling.

Now go and achieve all of your dreams!

**Visit
EmpowermentNation.com
to view other fantastic books,
sign up for book alerts, giveaways,
and updates!**